Contents

Seniors and Nutrition

Seniors and Nutrition

Judith Swarth, MS, RD

Publisher: Robert H. Garrison, Jr., MA, RPh

Editor In Chief: Elizabeth Somer, MA, RD

Managing Editor: Lisa M. Moye

Editorial Director: Janet L. Haley

Art Director: Scott Mayeda

Production Directors: Jeff Elkind, Irene Villa, Becky Moyer

Copy Editors: Norma Trost Foor, Jean Forsythe, Mary Houser, Stephen C. Schneider, R. H. Garrison, Sr.

Cover Design: Stefanko & Hetz, Jeff Elkind

Photography: Bob and Irene Nishihira, Carlsbad, CA

Illustration: Jennifer Hewitson, Julian Naranjo, Walter Stuart

For information regarding volume purchase discounts contact:
Health Media of America, Inc.
11300 Sorrento Valley Road, Suite 250
San Diego, CA 92121

Printed in the United States of America.

ISBN 0-937325-09-0

Introduction

Older and Wiser: Nutrition Is Important

"Aging begins with the moment of birth, and it ends only when life itself has ended. Old age is not a disease — it is strength and survivorship, triumph over all kinds of vicissitudes and disappointments, trials and illnesses." — Margaret E. Kahn, founder of the Gray Panthers.[1]

It is not unusual to read about 60 year old marathon runners or 60 year old heart surgery patients. The number of older adults in the United States is increasing, with one in every nine adults 65 years old or older.[2] This rapidly growing group has doubled in size in the last 50 years and is expected to increase from the current 27 million individuals to over 34 million individuals in the year 2010.[1] *(Graph 1)*

Graph 1. Percentage Of The U.S. Population 65 Years And Older.

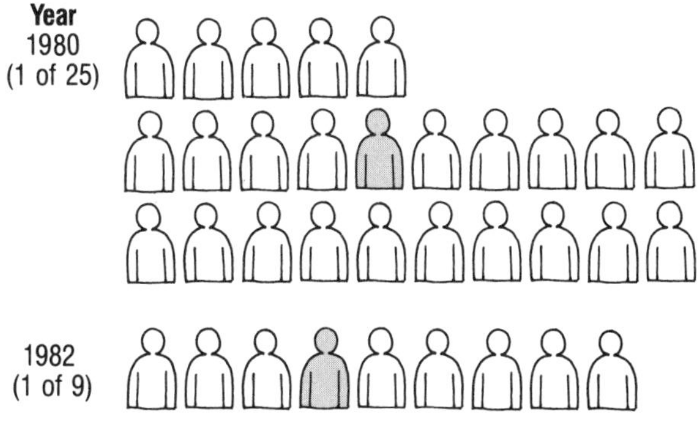

One out of every nine citizens in the United States is above 65 years of age, and the percentage is increasing.

The older years can be active and rewarding. Illness and poor health are not an inevitable part of growing older. Many of the degenerative diseases that affect millions of older adults, such as cardiovascular disease, cancer, stroke, osteoporosis, high blood pressure, and diabetes, are related to lifestyle and diet.[3]

Every part of the body undergoes natural changes with age, including the heart, lungs, brain, bones, muscles, skin, teeth, hair, eyes, and ears.[4] All cells in the body need a constant supply of vitamins, minerals, protein, and other nutrients to function throughout life. Adequate nutrition is important to prevent and treat illness and harmful changes in body tissues.

A person does not need to be a marathon runner to increase the chances for a long and healthy life. Simple changes in diet and exercise might prevent or treat several diseases and ensure the vitality and energy needed for an active body and alert mind. SENIORS AND NUTRITION will examine the many aspects of nutrition important to the health of body and mind of the older individual.

1
The Aging Process

Some researchers believe aging and death result from accumulated damage to cells over the years. This damage can be caused by toxic substances in the environment and in the diet, such as air pollution and some food preservatives. This damage can also be caused by toxins that result from normal body processes. According to this theory, the cells eventually stop functioning, organs become damaged, and death occurs.

Other researchers believe aging is determined by genetics.[1] The cells are programmed by the genetic code inside them to stop reproducing at a certain age and body systems slowly shut down until death occurs.

Stress accelerates the aging process. Stresses include very hot or cold climates, nutritional deficiencies, diseases, a sedentary (physically inactive) lifestyle, smoking, and a life of hard physical labor.[5,6]

Proper nutrition might be the best way to minimize the effects of aging and the associated illnesses.[7] Nutrition and other beneficial lifestyle habits reduce the effects of life's stresses and improve a person's chance for health and independence in later years.

The Changes Associated With Aging

The years have a subtle affect on the shape and function of the body. Although these changes are inevitable they might be slowed, or in some cases avoided, by proper nutrition and health care.

At the microscopic level, changes occur inside cells. Cells are the basic building blocks of organs, bones, skin, and other body tissues. Waste products of cellular activity accumulate inside cells over the years and might interfere with normal cell function.[4,8]

The genetic programming that regulates cell repair and regeneration becomes less efficient and cells misread their genetic material. As a result, cells produce the wrong molecules and body processes are impaired. Cells also stop reproducing themselves and some cells die.[4,8,9] In addition, cell membranes become more fragile. When the protective barrier of a cell membrane is damaged, substances can enter the cell and cause further damage.[1,4,8]

These changes in the health of individual cells affect organs and tissues. The body becomes less efficient in responding to hormones, the chemical messengers that regulate body processes.[4] Muscles in the small and large intestines weaken, blood vessels become stiff, the heart pumps less blood, and less blood flows to organs.[8] The kidneys filter fewer wastes and toxins from the blood and return fewer nutrients to it.

Fat is deposited in the liver, which hampers the liver's ability to work. Tissues draw fewer nutrients from the blood. The immune system weakens, which limits the body's defense against invading bacteria, viruses, and environmental toxins. The lungs hold less oxygen. Nerve signals relayed throughout the communication lines of the nervous system become more erratic.[8]

In older adults who do not exercise, muscle mass is gradually lost, more fat is stored, and bones weaken. Metabolism, which is all the physical and chemical changes that take place in the body, slows down by 12% to 20% in older adults.[10,11] Decreased metabolism reduces calorie needs.

The changes in tissues and organs affect body processes. Digestion of food depends on intestinal fluids and digestive enzymes, which are molecules that break apart food substances in the stomach and intestines. As a person ages, the quantity of digestive fluids and enzymes decreases. This can cause digestive upsets and poor absorption of nutrients.[10,12] In addition, the intestinal muscles are less efficient in later years and move food through the intestinal tract more slowly. Constipation can result.[8]

Changes in the nervous system impair eyesight and hearing.[4] Diminished senses of taste and smell make eating less pleasureable. Connective tissue is a substance that contributes to the tough, elastic quality of skin, tendons, blood vessels, and other tissues. As the body ages, connective tissues and skin become less elastic and gums are more susceptible to infection.[4] The gradual loss of nerve and brain cells might decrease mental capacities[9] and can cause memory loss and other behavior changes.[4,13]

Nutrition And The Aging Process: Obtaining Nourishment In The Later Years

The physical and mental changes of aging are not inevitable. A nutritious diet is important during this time of life. Poor nutrition might accelerate the aging process. One study of older adults showed that health was related to nutrient intake and that rates for illness and premature death were highest in people who consumed diets low in vitamins and minerals.[14]

Studies show that older adults do not obtain the necessary vitamins and minerals for health.[15,16]

Obtaining adequate nourishment is difficult for older persons. The reduction in digestion, taste, and smell and problems with teeth and gums contribute to the difficulty.

Many older persons are socially isolated or live alone. Social companionship is as important to good eating habits as the diet itself.[10] Shopping and preparing meals might be difficult for those with arthritis, physical weakness, or illness.[11] Seniors on fixed incomes might not buy nutritious food. Chronic illnesses, such as diabetes and kidney disease, require careful attention to diet that might be difficult for some people.

Elderly persons living in institutions might eat less if served foods they do not enjoy or if they are pressured to eat at designated times.[11] Many commonly-used drugs interfere with nutrients in the body.[17]

Malnutrition in older adults is a complex process that can include social, physical, emotional, and economic factors. A nutritious diet during the later years can prevent or treat malnutrition and might improve some physical, emotional, and even social factors associated with aging. *(Table 1, Page 5)*

Table 1 Possible Signs Of Nutritional Deficiencies In Older Adults

- Loss of appetite
- Loss of taste or smell
- Weight loss
- Weight gain
- Pain or discomfort when eating or swallowing
- Sore lips, tongue, or throat
- Vomiting
- Regurgitation of food
- Change in bowel habits
- Diarrhea
- Blood in the stools
- "Rash" (dermatitis) that does not respond to topical medication
- Bleeding skin or easy bruising
- Slow healing of wound, sore, or ulcer
- Changes in skin color (yellow, brown, grey)
- Light sensitivity
- Swelling of the legs
- Hair loss
- Thin nails
- Breathlessness on exertion and/or at rest
- Burning, pricking, pins and needles, or cramps in the legs
- Loss of balance
- Confusion
- Loss of memory
- Depression

2
Nutritional Needs Of Older Adults

How Well Nourished Are Older Adults?

The physical, emotional, and social demands of aging affect the nutritional needs of the older adult.

The diets of older adults are often low in several nutrients, including protein, vitamin A, vitamin C, vitamin B_1, vitamin B_2, niacin, folic acid, vitamin B_6, iron, calcium, and magnesium.[18-24] Other nutrients likely to be low are the trace minerals chromium and zinc.[25,26] Additionally, the adequacy of other minerals and trace elements has not been investigated. Also, older adults often do not consume adequate calories.[18]

Women are more likely than men to be deficient in calcium and iron and men are more likely to be deficient in vitamin C, especially if they eat few fruits and vegetables.[18] Those who do not eat several servings a day of fresh vegetables and fruit might be at risk for deficiencies of folic acid, vitamin A, and potassium.[27,28]

Older adults who limit their milk intake can lack adequate dietary calcium, vitamin B_2, and vitamin D.[27] Older persons who are not exposed to sunshine might not produce enough vitamin D to meet their needs. Unless fortified milk is consumed, they might be deficient in this fat-soluble vitamin and at greater risk for developing osteoporosis and tooth disorders.[29]

When consumption of whole grain breads and cereals is low, there might be chronic low intake of B vitamins and minerals.[8] Processed foods and convenience foods used by the elderly often are low in vitamin E and high in fats, sugars, and salt.[30] Evidence shows that the higher the intake of fat, the shorter the lifespan.[7]

One in four older women and one in five older men eat less than two-thirds of the calories they need for optimal health.[18,20,23] In contrast, one-half of older women and one-fifth of older men are obese and weigh 20% more than they should.[18] Undernutrition, too few calories, and nutrients; and obesity, too many calories, and inadequate exercise are the leading nutritional problems in older adults.

Nutritional Guidelines

Variety is the Spice of Life: Different foods are available throughout the year. These foods provide variety in color, shape, texture, smell, and taste. They also provide variety in nutrition.

No one food or food group contains all the nutrients essential to health. Milk and milk products such as cheese, yogurt, and buttermilk provide vitamin B_2, calcium, protein, and vitamin A. But these products are low in other nutrients such as iron. Lean meats, chicken, fresh fish, and dried beans and peas provide iron and protein, but are low in calcium and vitamin D. Because of the unique nutrient spectrums, daily servings from each food group are recommended. These groups are whole grain breads and cereals, fresh fruits and vegetables, lean meats and dried beans and peas, and low-fat milk and low-fat dairy products. *(Figure 1, Page 8)*

Figure 1. **Recommended Daily Foods From The Four Food Groups**

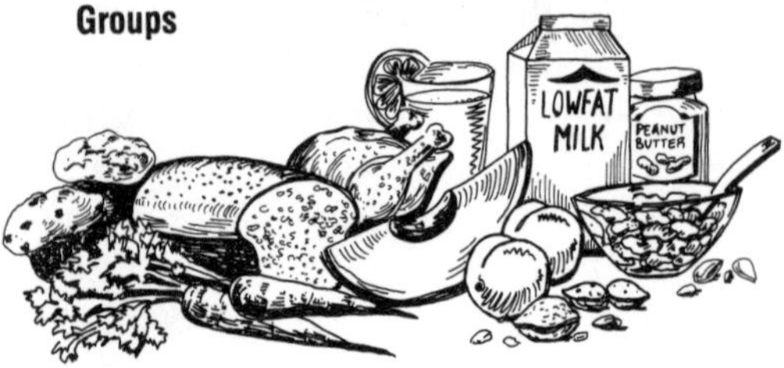

Group	Examples of Foods:	Servings	Household Measure
Dairy	Lowfat milk, lowfat cheese		16 oz.
or	American cheese	2	1 slice
Meat	Chicken +	1	3 oz.
	Peanut Butter	1	1 tbsp.
or	Lean beef, lamb, or veal +	1	3 oz.
	Dried beans and peans	1	½ cup
Vegetables and Fruit	Broccoli +	1	½ cup
	Tomatoes +	1	2 medium
	Orange juice	2	1½ cups
or	Carrots +	1	½ cup
	Spinach +	1	½ cup
	Cantaloupe +	1	½ cup
	Orange juice	1	¾ cup
Breads and Cereals	Bread, enriched or whole grain	3	3 slices
	Cold cereal, fortified	1	½ cup
or	Bran muffin +	2	2
	Rice, brown +	1	½ cup
	Bread, whole wheat	1	1 slice

Foods in the same group can contain different amounts of nutrients. Winter squash, for example, is much higher in vitamin A than summer squash. Strawberries are a good source of iron but contain little vitamin A; carrots are an excellent source of vitamin A but contain little vitamin C; and potatoes are a good source of vitamin C but contain little folic acid. Variety in the diet guarantees that all the vitamins and minerals will be supplied.

Variety makes the diet enjoyable. Meals are more interesting with different tastes, aromas, and textures. Senses of taste and smell diminish with age and new flavors can stimulate taste buds and improve food consumption in undereaters.

Whole and Unprocessed Foods: The closer foods are to their natural state, the more likely they are to contain more vitamins and minerals and less fat, salt, and sugar than processed varieties. A processed food is any food that is canned, frozen, dried, or otherwise treated or "refined."

This does not mean processed foods should never be eaten. Many processed foods are nutritious, such as dried nonfat milk, frozen orange juice, and frozen broccoli. Other processed foods, however, might have lost nutritional value during processing. For example, the high heat of canning destroys vitamin B_6, a nutrient low in many diets. White bread made with refined flour contains lower amounts of several vitamins and minerals as compared to whole wheat bread. White breads and white rice are also low in fiber, a dietary substance that prevents constipation and might reduce the risk for cancer, diabetes, and cardiovascular disease.

Many processed foods contain added fat, sugar, and salt. These nutrients are linked to an increased risk for developing cardiovascular disease, diabetes, hypertension, and obesity.[31] The lower calorie needs of the older person leaves less room for excess dietary fat and sugar.

A diet of whole and unprocessed foods contains several servings each day of fresh fruits and vegetables; dried beans and peas, lean meat, skinned chicken, or fish; whole grain breads and cereals; and low-fat milk and low-fat milk products.

Calories: Calories from food provide energy to the body. The body needs energy for processes such as the heartbeat, breathing, maintaining body temper ature, and physical activity. Calorie needs decline between the ages of 46 years old and 75 years old. An individual needs 200 fewer calories in the daily diet to maintain ideal weight. Calorie needs decrease even more past the late 70s, when a person needs 400 to 500 fewer calories daily than were required in younger years.[32] Calorie intake is balanced with energy needs if a person maintains a weight that approaches the ideal within five to ten pounds.

If a person consumes as much food as he or she did when younger, the result probably will be obesity. However, eating too little food can result in nutrient deficiencies. When calorie intake is less than 1,800 calories a day, the diet might be deficient in protein, calcium, iron, and vitamins.[24,33]

Protein, carbohydrates such as starches and sugars, fat, and alcohol all provide calories. Older persons can meet nutritional needs by avoiding foods and beverages high in fat, sugar, or alcohol that provide few vitamins and minerals. Emphasis can be placed on lower calorie but nutrient-rich foods such as whole grain breads and cereals, lean meat, fish and poultry, dried beans and peas, fruits, vegetables, and low-fat or nonfat milk products.

Protein: Protein is needed to maintain a strong immune system. Physical stress, such as illness or infection, increases protein needs.[27] If a person does not consume enough calories, some protein is burned for energy, rather than used to build and repair tissues.

Adequate protein intake is important to maintain health, but excesses of protein increase losses of calcium and other minerals from bone and add to the risk of developing osteoporosis. If kidney function is poor, extra protein strains these organs.[3,8]

Older people frequently consume inadequate amounts of protein-rich foods. In addition, protein needs might increase with age.[12] Low protein intake can contribute to edema, itching of the skin and related skin disorders, fatigue, muscle weakness, and loss of muscle.[24] Low protein intake is often associated with vitamin and mineral deficiencies.

The diet should include four servings a day from the protein-rich food groups, such as lean meats, fish, poultry, dried beans and peas, tofu (soy bean curd), eggs, low-fat milk, yogurt, low-fat cheese, and buttermilk. Breads, cereals, and other whole grains also contribute protein to the diet, especially if combined with low-fat milk, dried beans and peas, or nuts.

Dietary Fat: Although small amounts of fat in the diet are necessary for the absorption of the fat-soluble vitamins and for healthy skin and hair, the American diet is too high in fat.[31] This high fat intake is associated with an increased risk for cardiovascular disease, cancer, and other degenerative disorders.

Fat comes in three main forms: saturated, unsaturated, and cholesterol.

Saturated fats are found in foods from animal sources such as meat, milk, cheese and eggs, and in vegetable fats such as palm and coconut oil. Saturated fats also are found in margarines and hydrogenated vegetable shortenings.

Unsaturated fats are found in peanut and olive oils, and in other vegetable oils, such as safflower, soy, and corn oil. Unsaturated fats also are found in chicken and fish.

Cholesterol does not supply calories or add body weight. However, cholesterol is associated with an increased risk for developing cardiovascular disease and is found only in foods from animal sources such as eggs, whole milk, beef, pork, luncheon meats, butter, and sour cream.

No more than 30% and no less than 10% of calories should come from saturated or unsaturated fat to guarantee adequate fat intake without increasing the risk for disease. In addition to fatty meats, dairy foods, and oils, many pre-prepared convenience foods are high in fat, such as frozen entrees and frozen vegetables in sauce, luncheon meats, and bacon. Foods lower in fat include dried beans and peas, whole grain breads and cereals, fresh fruits and vegetables, low-fat dairy foods, and small amounts of lean meat, chicken, and fish. *(Figure 2, Page 13)*

How food is prepared can reduce or increase fat and calorie intake. Foods that are sauteed, fried, or served with sauces and gravies can contain as much as twice the calories from fat as foods baked, steamed, or broiled.

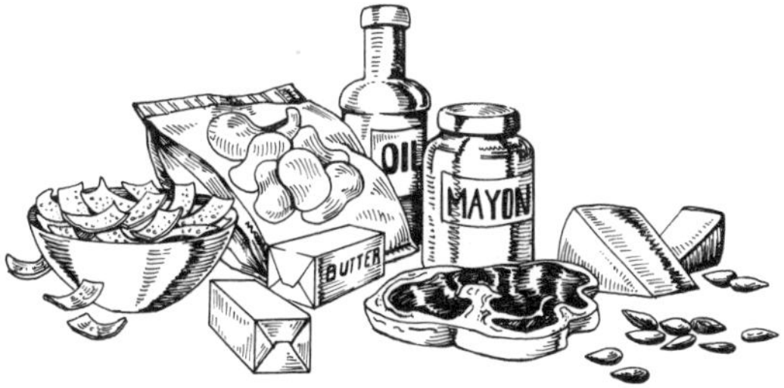

Figure 2. Foods High In Fat

To further reduce the fat in the diet:

- Limit portions of lean meats, chicken, and fish to 3 to 4 ounces, once or twice a day.
- Remove the skin before preparing chicken.
- Choose desserts that are low in fat, such as gelatin desserts, ice milk, angel food cake, or yogurt and fresh fruit.
- Choose salad dressings made with low-fat yogurt, nonfat cottage cheese, vinegar, lemon juice, or other seasonings rather than oil.

Vitamins And Minerals

Increasing the vitamin content of the diet might improve health.[24] Vitamins and minerals are important in all body processes. Several health concerns of older adults are related to poor vitamin and mineral intake. Poor intake is caused by a reduced capacity to digest and absorb vitamins and minerals; use of alcohol, or laxatives and other medications that reduce absorption or increase excretion of nutrients; and poor dietary habits. People with achlorhydria (low secretion of stomach acid) might not digest and absorb nutrients, such as iron. Evidence also suggests that changes occur with age that hinder the body's ability to use vitamins and minerals.[12,19-24]

Older adults are at risk for deficiencies of vitamin A, vitamin B_1, niacin, and vitamin C.[15] In a national nutrition survey, one-half of the men and three-quarters of the women did not meet their daily recommendation for vitamin A.[19] These deficiencies are associated with an increased risk for nervous, circulatory, and respiratory disorders.[7,15] These disorders might subside when the lacking nutrient is supplied in the diet. Eye disorders in older adults, such as night blindness, sometimes are corrected by inclusion of vitamin A-rich foods in the diet.[24,34]

Fatigue, confusion, disorientation, and depression are concerns of older adults. Poor absorption of vitamin B_{12} can result in marginal deficiencies of this nutrient and low blood levels of vitamin B_{12} are often found in the elderly popluation.[24] When vitamin B_{12} is added to the diet, many of these symptoms disappear.[35,36] Mental and behavioral disorders also respond to the inclusion of other B vitamins in the diet.[24]

A low intake of folic acid can cause anemia, poor concentration, and weakness. The likelihood of developing anemia increases with age.[37] Folic acid deficiency is found in older adults, especially those who do not consume a daily source of fresh dark green leafy vegetables.[24] Many medications commonly prescribed for older adults interfere with folic acid absorption and might encourage a deficiency.[38]

One of the most common symptoms of a mineral deficiency is osteoporosis and its associated risk for increased bone fractures and jaw bone degeneration.[39] Back bone degeneration caused by calcium loss from the bone is found in 80% of women more than 65 years old.[40] This bone loss begins in the 30s and progresses slowly throughout life. Poor dietary intake of calcium and limited exercise are linked to its progression.[41]

The best way to avoid vitamin and mineral deficiencies is to consume a varied diet of fresh, nutritious, foods. *(Figure 3, Page 16)* In addition, a multiple vitamin and mineral preparation that contains the recommended dietary allowance (RDA) for all vitamins and minerals might improve nutritional status, especially for persons eating less than 1,800 calories.[8,24]

Fiber: Fiber is the non-digestible portion of fruits, vegetables, dried beans and peas, and whole grain breads and cereals. Fiber includes a variety of substances including bran in whole wheat bread, pectin in apples and fruits, lignin in grains and dried beans, and dietary gums such as guar gum, which is a thickening agent added to foods.

Different fibers perform different functions in the body. A well-known benefit of wheat bran and the fiber in dried beans is their ability to prevent constipation. These fibers bind to water in the intestine and improve elimination. Fiber in wheat and beans might prevent diverticular disease, a condition of painful, inflammed pockets in the walls of the colon.[42] Fibers such as pectin, oat bran, and guar gum might reduce blood cholesterol levels.[43]

Figure 3. Major Nutrients Supplied By Different Food Groups

Food Group	Nutrients
Fruits and vegetables 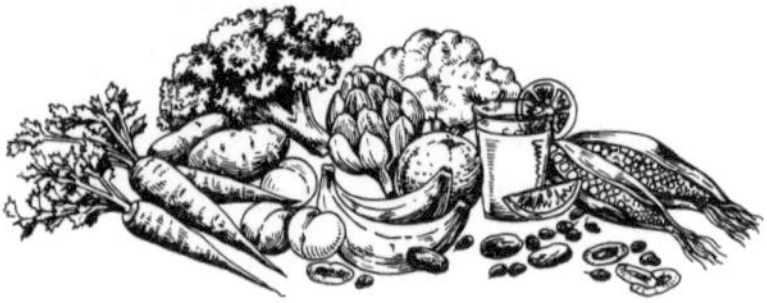	Vitamin A Vitamin C Folic Acid Trace minerals Potassium Fiber
Whole grain breads and cereals 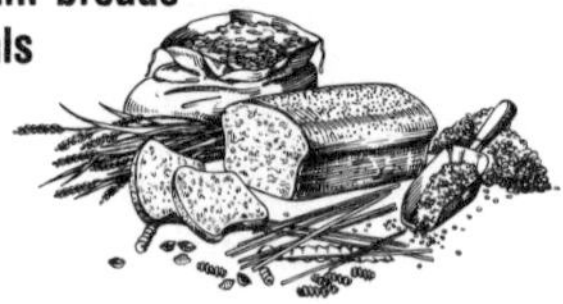	Protein B vitamins Trace minerals Fiber
Low-fat dairy foods 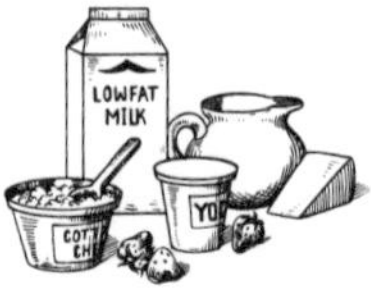	Protein Calcium Vitamin D (milk) Vitamin B2 Magnesium
Lean meats, chicken, fish, dried beans and peas 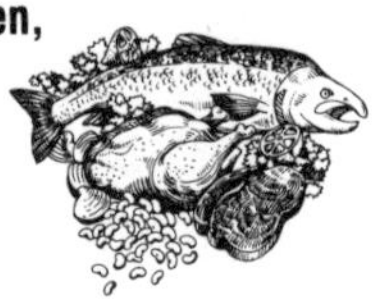	Protein B vitamins Trace minerals

Whole wheat bread, whole grains such as brown rice and oatmeal, bran flake cereals, dried beans and peas, and fresh fruits and vegetables are sources of fiber. Fiber is lost when grains are refined. Meats, fats, sugar, fruit juices, milk, eggs, and cheese are low in fiber.

Commercial bran products are high in fiber, but contain only one or two of the several types of fiber necessary for health. Too much fiber in the diet can interfere with the absorption of some minerals such as calcium, zinc, magnesium, and iron.[44] This is not a problem unless large amounts of commercial bran are consumed.[45]

Recommendations for fiber intake have not been established, but it is generally accepted that a diet that contains about 37 grams of fiber is beneficial to the health of all adults. This amount can be obtained from daily servings of the following:[46]

- 6 servings of whole grain breads and cereals (1 serving = 1 slice of bread or 1/2 cup cooked cereal or pasta) ....13 grams
- 4 servings of fresh fruits and vegetables (1 serving = 1 piece of fruit or vegetable, 1/2 cup cooked, or 1 cup raw) ....15-23 grams
- 1 serving of dried beans or peas (1 serving = 1/2 cup cooked)...........................9 grams

Total ....37-45 grams

Fluids: All body cells and organs need water to function. The blood needs water to maintain its volume. Water prevents overheating during exercise and the kidneys require water to flush wastes out in the urine. Adequate water helps prevent constipation and maintains moist skin and healthy hair.

The healthy adult needs about 6 to 8 glasses of water a day to maintain fluid balance.[47] In addition, low-fat milk, soups, and fruit and vegetable juices are good sources of fluid. Some bottled mineral waters and club sodas are high in sodium and might need to be avoided on salt-restricted diets.[48] Coffee, tea, and alcohol have a diuretic effect on the body and increase urinary exretion of fluids. They should not be considered part of the daily requirement for water.

Sugar: Sugar is a refined carbohydrate that provides calories, but does not provide vitamins or minerals. Because sugar requires several nutrients in order to be digested and used by the body, it uses more nutrients than it supplies.

Sugar is easily recognized as an ingredient in desserts, but its presence in other foods, such as canned and convenience foods and cereals, might go undetected. For example, catsup is 30% sugar.

For the older person with low caloric needs, there is little room in the diet for sweets. No more than 10% of calories should come from sugar.[31] In a diet of 2,000 calories, this allows one small dessert and a tablespoon of jam, honey, sugar, or other concentrated sweet. Jam, honey, and sugar should be used sparingly and sweet desserts should be consumed infrequently.

Caffeine: Caffeine stimulates the nervous system, improves concentration, and alters energy levels. Caffeine is found in coffee, black teas, cocoa and chocolate, soft drinks, and medications such as nonprescription pain relievers, appetite suppressants, and cold remedies. A person becomes more sensitive to caffeine with age and an excessive intake can cause jittery nerves, heart palpitations, or sleep problems.[8] A sudden decrease in caffeine intake can cause headaches and fatigue. These symptoms can be avoided by a gradual reduction in caffeine intake. Instant cereal beverages, decaffeinated coffee and tea, low-fat milk, and fruit and vegetable juices are all good substitutes for caffiene-containing beverages. *(Table 2)*

Alcohol: For some people, a glass of wine might aid in relaxation and help digestion. Too much alcohol, however, affects overall health. Alcohol reduces the absorption of several nutrients, interferes with

Table 2 Caffeine Content Of Selected Beverages, Foods, And Medications

Item	Milligrams Caffeine
Coffee (5 oz. cup), brewed, drip method	115
Tea (5 oz. cup), brewed	40
Cocoa beverage (5 oz. cup)	4
Milk chocolate (1 oz.)	6
Dark chocolate, semi-sweet (1 oz.)	20
Soft drinks (12 oz. serving)	30.0-58.8
Prescription Drugs	
Soma Compound (pain relief)	32
Darvon Compound (pain relief)	32.4
Nonprescription Drugs	
Weight-control aids	140-200
Alertness Tablets	100-200
Analgesic/Pain Relief	32-65
Diuretics	100-200
Cold/Allergy Remedies	16.2-30

Source: FDA, Food Additives Chemistry Evaluation Branch, based on evaluations of existing literature on caffeine levels.

use of other nutrients, and increases nutrient losses. Nutrients that are likely to be depleted because of alcohol use include vitamin C, vitamin B_1, vitamin B_2, niacin, vitamin B_6, vitamin B_{12}, folic acid, magnesium, zinc, calcium, and potassium.[49,50]

Alcohol provides calories, supplies no vitamins or minerals, and depresses appetite. It irritates the digestive tract and increases levels of fats in the blood. If consumed in excess, alcohol can cause liver disease.[50] *(Table 3, Page 21)*

Planning The Diet: A Summary

Guidelines for healthy eating must be individualized to meet the nutrient needs of each person.

A nutritious diet consists primarily of fresh fruits and vegetables, whole grain breads and cereals, and dried beans and peas, with at least two servings daily of lean meat, chicken, or fish and two servings of low-fat dairy foods. If fewer than 1,800 calories are consumed each day, a multiple vitamin and mineral supplement might be necessary to meet nutrient needs.

Dentures can limit the type and consistency of foods consumed. Foods such as fiberous vegetables can be mashed, chopped, strained, or pureed; sandwiches and lean meats can be cut into small pieces; and fruits can be sliced or lightly steamed for easy chewing.

If low-fat milk products are not well-tolerated another dietary or supplemental source of calcium and vitamin D must be found. Good sources of calcium include broccoli and dark green leafy vegetables; however, several cups must be consumed to equal the amount of calcium in two servings of low-fat milk. A

Table 3	Calories In Alcohol And Mixes		
	Beverage	**Amount**	**Calories**
	Beer	12 oz.	140-150
	Light Beer	12 oz.	95
	Dry Wine	3½ oz.	87
	Gin	1½ oz.	97
	Rum	1½ oz.	97
	Vodka	1½ oz.	97
	Whiskey	1½ oz.	97
	Brandy	1½ oz.	97
	Mixes		
	Club soda	8 oz.	0
	Ginger ale	8 oz.	72
	Cola	8 oz.	96
	Collins	8 oz.	112

supplement that provides no more than 400IU of vitamin D might be necessary if milk is avoided.

If a person has digestive problems, food is less likely to irritate the system if several small meals are consumed rather than three large meals, a warm to hot food is included at each meal, and the largest meal of the day is at lunch rather than dinner.

3
Nutrition And Special Concerns

Anemia

The main function of the red blood cells is to carry oxygen to the tissues. Within each red blood cell is a protein called hemoglobin that contains iron. The iron in red blood cells binds to oxygen in the lungs and carries it to the brain, heart, muscles, and other tissues. When a person is anemic, the production of red blood cells is reduced and the tissues do not receive an adequate amount of oxygen. The result is fatigue, poor concentration, anxiety, an increased susceptibility to colds and infections, and reduced appetite.

Several dietary factors contribute to anemia, including deficiencies of protein, vitamin C, vitamin B_6, vitamin B_{12}, folic acid, vitamin E, iron, and copper.[13,33,51,52]

Iron deficiency anemia commonly results from lack of iron in the diet. Foods high in iron are lean meat, dark green leafy vegetables, dried beans and peas, dried fruit, potatoes, and whole grain breads and cereals. Diets low in calories are likely to be iron-deficient. Vitamin C-rich foods increase absorption of iron and should be consumed often with meals. Some substances in foods interfere with iron absorption, including the tannins in tea, oxalates in chard, and a compound in eggs.[4] *(Figure 4, Page 23)*

Figure 4. Foods High In Iron

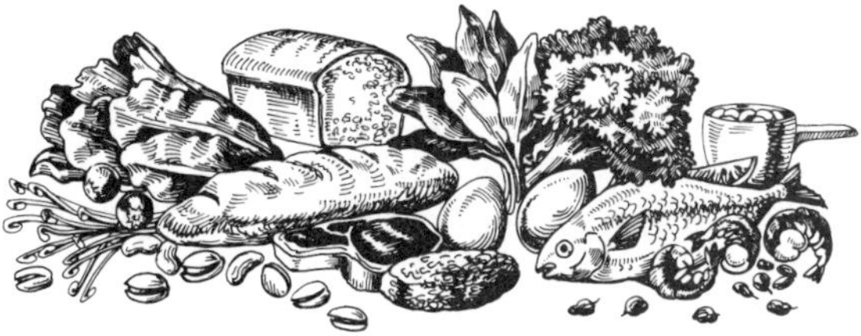

Meats	Non-Meat
Hamburger, cooked, lean	Filberts (hazelnuts)
Lamb chop, broiled	Pistachios
Shrimp	Cashews
Chicken breast, roasted	Whole-wheat bread
Perch	Enriched white bread
	Pinto beans, boiled
	Spinach, raw
	Raisins, seeded (Muscat)
	Eggs
	Bean sprouts
	Broccoli
	Romaine lettuce

Folic acid deficiency is also common.[52] Good sources of this B vitamin are dark green leafy vegetables (especially raw, since heat destroys folic acid), liver, asparagus, beets, legumes, citrus fruits, and whole grain breads and cereals.

Anemia from vitamin B_{12} deficiency can occur in older adults because of a reduced ability to absorb the vitamin. A substance in stomach juices needed for B_{12} absorption is produced in lesser quantities as a person ages and less vitamin B_{12} can be absorbed from the diet. Ample intake of vitamin B_{12} is important to guarantee adequate absorption.

Arthritis and Gout

Rheumatoid Arthritis: Rheumatoid arthritis is an autoimmune disease, meaning the body attacks its own tissues. This results in inflammation and swelling in the linings of joints, stiffness, and pain. Although any joint can be affected, those of the hands and feet are most often involved. With time, tissue surrounding bones and tendons is destroyed. This leads to crippling deformities and difficulty with movement.

A disturbed immune system, infection, and genetics might be involved in the development of the disease. Nutrition also might be involved.[53] The pain and stiffness of arthritis increase when a person is malnourished and improve when a person consumes a nutritious diet.[54]

Malnutrition is common in people with rhuematoid arthritis.[54] The inflammation of arthritis increases nutrient needs but lowers uptake of nutrients from the digestive tract. People with arthritis also have a difficult time preparing and shopping for food. In addition, steroid drugs used in treatment of arthritis cause calcium loss from the bones, which increases daily requirements for calcium and vitamin D to prevent osteoporosis.[55] Regular use of aspirin to reduce inflammation interferes with vitamin C in the body and might cause gastric bleeding that can lead to iron deficiency and anemia.[56] Because of the interaction between aspirin and vitamin C, they should be taken at different times of the day.

Deficiencies of vitamin C, folic acid, vitamin D, iron, zinc, and vitamin B_6 occur in people with arthritis.[57-61] Vitamin E and selenium might be beneficial in the treatment of this disorder.[62-63]

Many of these vitamins and minerals are important to a healthy immune system. A well-functioning immune system might be important in the prevention or treatment of rheumatoid arthritis. Nutrients particularly important are calories and protein, zinc, iron, copper, selenium, vitamin A, vitamin E, vitamin B_6, and folic acid.[64]

Dietary fat also might influence arthritis. Different types and amounts of fat in the diet affect levels of prostaglandins. Prostaglandins are hormone-like substances involved in the regulation of many body processes, including inflammation and immunity. The fat EPA *(See page 33)* might reduce levels of prostaglandins that cause inflammation.[65,72]

A nutritious diet is important in the treatment of rheumatoid arthritis. Adequate intake of all vitamins and minerals improves a person's defense against disease and might reduce pain and stiffness.[66-73]

Gout: Gout is the accumulation of uric acid crystals in and near joints. This accumulation causes swelling, inflammation, and pain. The likelihood of developing gout increases with age and is more common in men than women. Effective medications are available that flush uric acid from the body and help prevent attacks. A person with gout should consult a physician about proper therapy for this disorder.

For those with moderate to high levels of uric acid in the blood, dietary measures might help. Maintenance of proper weight can reduce a person's risk for developing gout. Alcohol raises uric acid levels, and gout sufferers should reduce or eliminate alcoholic beverages.[74,75] Uric acid is formed from compounds called purines found in some protein foods.[76] Organ meats, sardines, mackerel, herring, and anchovies are especially high in purines.

Other meats, dried beans and peas, and fish contain lesser amounts. Low-fat dairy foods, fruits, and vegetables are low in purines. Nutritional or brewer's yeast, fat, and sugar also increase uric acid levels.

Behavior And Nutrition: Nutrition plays a role in a healthy mind as well as a healthy body. It has been known for decades that an extreme deficiency of certain nutrients, such as vitamin B_1 and niacin, results in severe mental problems. New research indicates that marginal deficiencies also affect a person's mental state.

Depression is not always related to nutritional habits; however, some nutritional causes of depression might include deficiencies of niacin, thiamin, or folic acid.[77,78]

In recent years identification of a substance in the brain called serotonin has linked nutrition to sleep, appetite, and mood. Both high protein meals and low vitamin B_6 in the diet might reduce serotonin formation and cause sleep difficulties and depression. Serotonin levels increase and depression might disappear in some cases following supplementation with vitamin B_6.[79,80] Low levels of serotonin are found in some suicidal patients.[81,82] *(Figure 5, Page 27)*

Vitamin B_6 is found in protein-rich foods such as lean meats, fish, poultry, legumes, and whole grain breads and cereals. Refined white bread and canned foods contain little of the vitamin. Vitamin B_6 might cause nerve damage when taken at doses greater than 500 mg.[83]

The calming action of serotonin affects sleep patterns as well. In addition to vitamin B_6, serotonin formation requires tryptophan. Tryptophan is an amino acid, one of the building blocks of protein. Supplements of tryptophan combined with a high-

Figure 5. Diet Might Affect Behavior

In recent years identification of a substance in the brain called serotonin has linked nutrition to sleep, appetite, and mood.

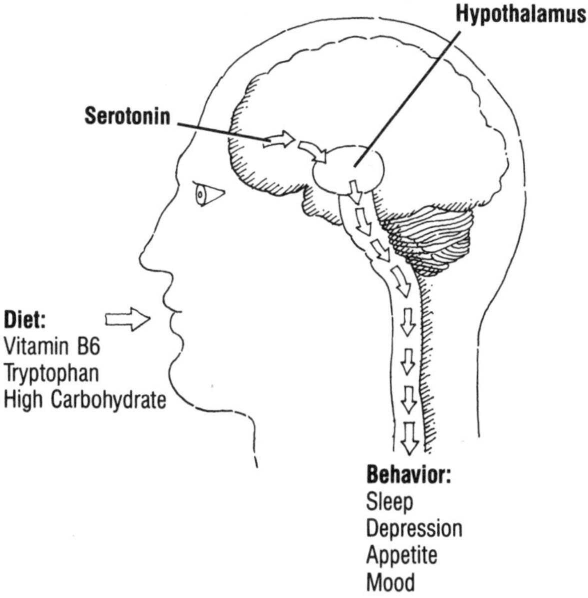

carbohydrate, low-protein meal might produce a calming effect that enables people to fall asleep easily.[84,85]

Memory also is affected by nutrition. Lack of vitamin B_{12} is associated with poor memory in the elderly.[85,86] Impaired memory can be an early sign of the severe, progressive senility of Alzheimer's disease. Choline is a vitamin-like substance found in dried beans and peas, wheat germ, and organ meats that might be important in the health of the nerves involved in memory.[87] The metal aluminum might interfere with reactions in nerve cells involving choline and be involved in development of Alzheimer's disease.[88] Adequate dietary calcium might prevent the accumulation of aluminum.

Bones

Bones deteriorate when the diet is low in calcium and a person is sedentary. Over the years, the daily loss of calcium from the bones can result in osteoporosis. By age 70 many women have lost half of their bone mass and 40% of women have experienced spontaneous fractures. Fractures heal poorly in the elderly, especially when the elderly are malnourished. Fractures can lead to infections and disability.[89-91]

Factors that contribute to bone loss include lack of exercise, hormonal changes after menopause (decreased estrogen), and dietary deficiencies.[92] Nutrients needed to maintain healthy bones include calcium, vitamin D, phosphorus, magnesium, and flouride.[93,94] Cigarette smoking, alcohol, caffeine, and excess protein and phosphorus are associated with thinning bones.[89]

The recommendation for calcium is 1,000 to 1,500 mg a day to prevent bone loss.[95-98] This is above the 500 mg most women consume or the 800 mg suggested by the RDA.[99,100] As a person ages, calcium is absorbed less efficiently from the digestive tract, which increases the importance of an ample intake of the mineral daily.[101] An increased intake of calcium might not only prevent osteoporosis, but also might help regenerate some lost bone tissue.[102] *(Table 4, Page 29)*

Table 4 Foods High In Calcium

Food	Weight or Measure	Calcium (Milligrams)
Plain nonfat and low-fat yogurts	1 cup	350-450
Dry nonfat milk	¼ cup	350-450
Nonfat and low-fat milks	1 cup	250-350
Swiss cheese	1 ounce	250-350
Hard cheeses such as Cheddar and Edam	1 ounce	150-250
Salmon, with bones	3 ounces	150-250
Collard greens	½ cup	150-250
Soft cheeses such as mozzarella, blue and feta	1 ounce	50-150
Cooked dried beans such as navy, pea, and lima	1 cup	50-150
Turnip greens, kale, dandelion greens	½ cup	50-150
Cottage cheeses	½ cup	50-150
Broccoli	½ cup	50-150
Orange	1 fresh	50-150
Dates, raisins	¼ cup	20-50
Bread, whole-wheat	1 slice	20-50
Cabbage	½ cup	20-50

Vitamin D also protects against bone losses.[103,104] Vitamin D deficiency is associated with soft bones, a condition called osteomalacia.[105] Inadequate exposure to sunlight combined with aging kidneys that are less capable of manufacturing vitamin D can place an older person at risk for a vitamin D deficiency unless dietary sources are adequate.[106] The only reliable source of vitamin D is vitamin D-fortified milk; other dairy products are not fortified with the vitamin. The RDA for vitamin D (400 IU) can be obtained each day from one quart of milk, by frequent exposure to sunlight, or through supplements. Vitamin D can be toxic and no more than three times the RDA should be consumed on a regular basis.[104,107]

Regular exercise is important to the maintenance of healthy bones.[108] Exercise such as walking, jogging, or jumping rope puts pressure on the bones and increases the deposition of calcium into bones, which thickens and stengthens these tissues.

Cancer And Nutrition

Many forms of cancer are affected by diet. Between 35% and 60% of cancers are thought to be related to diet.[109] Cancer of the breast, colon, uterus, ovaries, and prostate are linked to low-fiber and high-fat consumption.[110] Besides fat and fiber, other dietary components are related to cancer.

Vitamin C, vitamin E, and selenium are nutrients that protect cells from damage and possible cancer. These nutrients either protect cell membranes from damage from highly reactive compounds called free radicals that might initiate cancer or they inhibit the formation of cancer-causing substances.

Consumption of vitamin C-rich foods is associated with a lower incidence of stomach and esophageal cancer.[111,112] In addition to protecting cell membranes, vitamin C neutralizes some substances in food that might promote cancer. Vitamin C is also essential to a healthy immune system, which might defend the body against cancer-causing agents.[113,114]

Vitamin E protects tissues from cancer-causing free radicals in polluted air and cigarette smoke.[115] Vitamin E also might inhibit the growth of certain tumors.[116,117]

Selenium works with vitamin E to protect cell membranes. Selenium also might strengthen the immune system.[118] Patients with cervical and endometrial cancers are found to have low blood levels of selenium.[119] The amount of selenium in the diet depends on the selenium content of the soil in which the food is grown.[120,121] Seafood, meat, poultry, eggs, and whole grains are the most reliable sources of selenium.

Another nutrient that might protect a person from developing cancer is vitamin A. Two forms of vitamin A exist. Retinol is the active form of vitamin A found in foods from animal sources such as organ meats, eggs, and milk products. Foods from plant sources contain beta-carotene, which is converted into vitamin A in the body. A diet high in beta-carotene-rich fruits and vegetables appears to decrease the risk of lung cancer.[122-124] Several studies show a relationship between vitamin A intake and a reduced incidence or growth of cancers.[125-130]

The form of vitamin A found in foods from animal sources and some supplements is toxic in large doses. Liver damage, skin and bone problems, headaches, and even death can occur if very large doses are taken over long periods of time.[131,132] Beta-carotene, the source of vitamin A found in plants, is not toxic, although large doses will temporarily turn the skin yellow.[131] consume two or more servings of foods rich in beta carotene each day. Dark green leafy vegetables and deep yellow and orange fruits and vegetables are high in beta-carotene.

Vegetables in the cabbage family might protect an individual from developing cancer. The Committee on Diet, Nutrition and Cancer of the National Research Council recommends frequent consumption of cabbage, broccoli, cauliflower, and Brussels sprouts.

Consumption of smoked and cured meats, salt-cured foods, pickled foods and alcohol, all of which contribute to cancer risk, should be limited.[109]

Cardiovascular Disease

Cardiovascular disease (CVD) is the major cause of death in the United States and it is linked to diet and lifestyle. Several factors are involved in the development of CVD including family history of heart disease, male gender, smoking, diabetes, overweight, stress, lack of exercise, high blood pressure, and a diet high in saturated fat and cholesterol.

Blood flow is reduced and the oxygen and nutrient supply to the tissues declines when fatty deposits of cholesterol build up in blood vessels. This process is called atherosclerosis. High amounts of cholesterol in the blood are associated with an increased risk for developing atherosclerosis. The clogged blood vessels in this disease increase the likelihood of a heart attack or stroke.

A diet high in fiber and complex carbohydrates and low in fat and sugar lowers blood levels of cholesterol and might prevent or slow the atherosclerotic process.

It is never too late to make changes in diet and exercise habits that can reduce the likelihood of developing CVD. The U.S. Dietary Goals recommend that people consume no more than 30% of their calories as fat and no more than 300 mg of cholesterol a day. Sugar should account for only 10% of the total calories and starchy foods should provide the major contribution to the diet.[31]

One dietary fat might protect an individual from developing CVD. Eicosapentaenoic acid (EPA) is a polyunsaturated fat found in fish. EPA might lower blood cholesterol and reduce the risk for developing CVD.[133,134] Several servings a week of EPA-rich foods such as salmon, mackerel, sardines, and codfish would provide a good supply of EPA.

Some types of fiber lower cholesterol and reduce the risk for developing CVD.[135] Oatmeal, fruits, vegetables, and dried beans and peas contain the type of fiber that can lower cholesterol. A diet composed of whole, unprocessed foods such as fresh fruits and vegetables, dried beans and peas, whole grain breads and cereals, and low-fat milk products provides the best dietary health protection from CVD.

High Blood Pressure: One in every five people develops hypertension (high blood pressure) and one in every two people age 65 to 75 years old suffers from it.[136] Hypertension increases the risk of developing CVD and kidney disease.

The best prevention against hypertension is to reduce the amount of salt and fat in the diet, maintain normal body weight, and consume an adequate amount of calcium.[137,138] Often a reduction in weight alone lowers blood pressure.[56] Calcium supplements can lower blood pressure in some individuals.[139] Adequate intake of potassium and a reduction in salt also might reduce blood pressure.[140] A diet low in total fat with a greater amount of fat from vegetable oils than from foods from animal sources might lower blood pressure.[141-145] *(Figure 6)*

Figure 6. Sodium Content Of Selected Food (in mg)

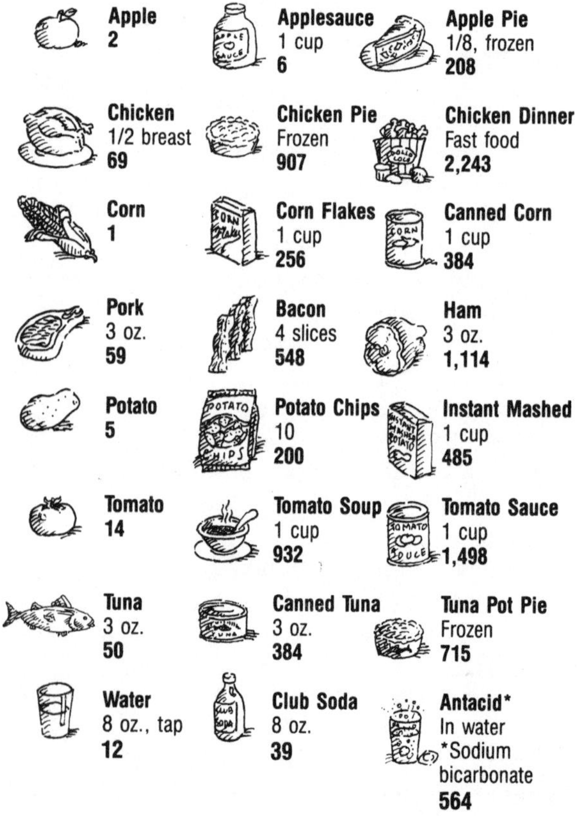
Apple
2
Applesauce
1 cup
6
Apple Pie
1/8, frozen
208
Chicken
1/2 breast
69
Chicken Pie
Frozen
907
Chicken Dinner
Fast food
2,243
Corn
1
Corn Flakes
1 cup
256
Canned Corn
1 cup
384
Pork
3 oz.
59
Bacon
4 slices
548
Ham
3 oz.
1,114
Potato
5
Potato Chips
10
200
Instant Mashed
1 cup
485
Tomato
14
Tomato Soup
1 cup
932
Tomato Sauce
1 cup
1,498
Tuna
3 oz.
50
Canned Tuna
3 oz.
384
Tuna Pot Pie
Frozen
715
Water
8 oz., tap
12
Club Soda
8 oz.
39
Antacid*
In water
*Sodium bicarbonate
564

Colds And Infections

Infections and colds can increase in the elderly, especially if disease is present.[146,147] The immune system responds less efficiently with age.[4] Nutrition is important in strengthening the immune system. Nutrients of particular importance are protein, the vitamin B complex, vitamin C, vitamin A, vitamin E, iron, copper, selenium, and zinc. A nutritious diet of unprocessed foods from all the food groups is essential to protect against colds and infections. Equally important is consuming enough calories, since one of the most common forms of malnutrition in older adults is inadequate calorie intake.[64]

Diabetes

Incidence of diabetes is high among the elderly, with 15% to 20% affected.[148] In diabetes, glucose levels in the blood are high because glucose cannot enter the tissues. In addition to depriving the tissues of energy, high blood glucose causes severe health complications, including kidney disease, impaired vision, cataracts, and heart disease.[149-152]

Controlling blood sugar levels is important in older adults to prevent the serious health effects of diabetes. Most adult diabetics can control blood glucose levels with oral medications and diet.[152] For many seniors, however, dietary control is difficult. Arthritis, tremors, and physical weakness make it hard to shop for and prepare food. Eating is difficult with dental problems and diminished senses of taste, smell, and sight make eating less pleasureable.

All these factors contribute to poor eating habits. Poor kidney function, infections, cancer, medications, and physical inactivity all upset the blood sugar balance.[152,153]

Most people who develop diabetes later in life are overweight. Weight reduction is the first and most important step in controlling adult-onset diabetes.[152] A healthy body weight often returns glucose metabolism to normal and no other measures are needed. In other cases a nutritious diet high in fiber and complex carbohydrates (starch) is needed.[154] Both fiber and complex carbohydrates help stabilize blood glucose. Since concentrated sweets do the opposite they need to be limited.

Adequate dietary chromium (50ug to 200ug/day) helps regulate blood sugar and might be an effective aid in the treatment for adult-onset diabetes.[155,156] Good sources of chromium include whole wheat bread and whole grain cereals, brown rice, vegetables, and nutritional yeast. High chromium yeast supplements are also available.

Digestive Disturbances

The digestive processes can slow as a person ages. Adjustments in nutritional habits are important to reduce discomfort and avoid health problems. Serious health conditions can mimic common digestive disorders; gallbladder disease, hiatal hernias, spastic colon, colitis (inflammation of the colon), and ulcers can produce feelings and symptoms similar to simple digestive disturbances. If digestive upsets persist, a physician should be consulted.

Constipation: Many people suffer from constipation at one time or another. Frequent occurrence is both uncomfortable and leads to more serious problems, such as hemmorhoids and diverticular disease. A diet that consists of processed and refined foods, such as white breads and cereals, white rice, and sugary foods, and is low in fresh fruits, vegetables, and dried beans and peas can contribute to chronic constipation in older adults.

A high-fiber and low-fat diet is essential to avoid constipation.[1,157] The type of fiber found in whole wheat bread and whole grain cereals is most effective.[158] Bran or oat bran sprinkled on cereal, or added to soups, stews, and casseroles can help relieve symptoms of constipation. Fiber from vegetables such as carrots, celery, and potatoes also is useful. Fluid consumption should be increased. Fresh fruits and vegetables add both fiber and fluid to the diet. A glass of prune juice, lemon juice in warm water, or other warm drink in the morning might be helpful.

In addition to diet, exercise improves muscle tone and the muscular activity of the digestive tract. Moderate physical activity such as daily walks improves digestive problems.[158,56]

Overuse of laxatives is common among older adults and can be harmful.[159] The laxative mineral oil binds to the fat-soluble vitamins A, D, E, and K in the intestine and increases their excretion. Mineral oil can cause deficiency of vitamin D, which contributes to the brittle bones of osteoporosis. Vitamin A deficiency adds to risk of cancer, poor eyesight, and skin problems. Lack of vitamin K leads to easy bruising and bleeding problems.[33]

Because of the potential for dependency on laxatives, treatment for constipation should combine a high-fiber diet, plenty of fluids, and regular exercise.

Individuals should avoid chronic use of laxatives. If constipation persists, a physician should be consulted.

Heartburn: Heartburn is a burning, uncomfortable sensation in the middle chest that occurs after meals. The heart itself is not involved, but rather the esophagus, which is the passageway between the throat and stomach. A small muscle at the bottom of the esophagus, called the sphincter, weakens and acidic stomach juices backflow into the esophagus. Some foods cause the sphincter muscle to open. These include spearmint and peppermint, coffee (regular and decaffeinated), fatty and fried foods, spicy foods, peppers, tomatoes, salad dressings, tomato and orange juices, radishes, and alcohol. Overeating and smoking a cigarette after meals also leads to heartburn.[160]

Heartburn can be controlled by eating small meals low in fat and high in both protein and carbohydrate. Maintenance of ideal weight can reduce the pressure placed on the muscle that leads to the esophagus and might improve symptoms of heartburn.[160]

Flatulence: The formation of excessive gas is caused by the following:

1. swallowing air while eating,
2. increased rate of movement of food in the intestine, or
3. excessive bacterial digestion of foods in the intestine.

Eating while relaxed and taking time to thoroughly chew food can reduce the amount of air swallowed.

A sudden increase in fiberous foods in the diet can speed the transport of undigested products through the intestine. The normal production of gases during the digestion of foods is usually absorbed through the walls of the intestine and dispersed in the blood. But when foods move too quickly through the intestinal tract these gases do not have time to disperse. A gradual increase in fiber intake over a few weeks allows the intestines time to adapt and might reduce the formation of intestinal gases.[161]

Adults with intolerance to the milk sugar lactose experience gas if they drink milk. This is a result of undigested milk sugar being broken down by bacteria in the intestine and the production of gases. Small amounts of milk often can be tolerated without discomfort.

Several foods can increase the production of intestinal gas including carbonated beverages, whipped cream, dried beans and peas, cabbage, onions, and wheat. The gas-producing potential of beans is reduced by soaking them before cooking, discarding the water, and consuming these foods in small amounts.

Diverticulosis: A diet adequate in fiber also appears to prevent diverticulosis, a condition in which small pockets protrude from the colon wall and become infected and inflammed. Diverticulosis is common in affluent, industrialized countries where the diet is high in meat, fat, and sugar and low in fiber. People from countries with low rates of these diseases develop them within two generations after they migrate to the United States and consume the typical American diet.[162]

Diverticulosis seldom develops before age 40, which suggests that the results of a low-fiber diet takes years to develop. Excessive pressure from constipation causes pouches in the intestinal wall to develop. In contrast, fiber increases the size of the stool. This expands the diameter of the colon, reduces pressure in the colon wall, and prevents diverticulosis from developing.[163]

Colon Cancer: A low-fiber, high-fat diet might contribute to the risk for developing colon cancer. People who consume low-fat diets have low rates of colon cancer.[163-167] In response to a high-fat meal, bile is released into the intestine. Though useful for digestion, bile also might generate cancer-causing substances in the intestine. Excessive dietary fat stimulates increased secretion of bile after a meal and might increase the risk for cancer. Fat also might encourage the growth of cancer-causing bacteria in the intestine.[168]

Fiber is also useful in the prevention of cancer. Some bacteria in the intestine produce cancer-causing substances. Fiber dilutes the contents of the intestine and reduces the effects of cancer-causing substances. Fiber also binds bile and lessens its cancerous effects. Like fat, fiber influences the bacteria in the colon, but while fat promotes harmful populations of bacteria, fiber promotes beneficial ones.[169]

Oral Health

Several factors related to oral health can interfere with proper nutrition.[170,171] For example, osteoarthritis in the jaw and gum inflammation from poorly fitting dentures can make chewing difficult.[4] Osteoporosis and smoking both contribute to loss of teeth and by age 65, half of Americans have lost their teeth.[10,172] To retard loss of calcium from the jaw bone and reduce the risk for loss of teeth, the diet should contain ample amounts of calcium, vitamin D, magnesium, and protein.

For people with poor-fitting dentures or lost teeth, vegetables, fruits, nuts, and lean meats can be difficult to chew. These foods are excellent sources of fiber, protein, vitamins, and minerals and their inclusion in the diet is important to health and the prevention of disease. These foods can be cooked, chopped, pureed, included in soups and stews, or cut into small bite-sized pieces for easy chewing.[173]

Taste and smell diminish over the years and food might taste bland, bitter, or sour.[174-177] A zinc deficiency also can cause changes in taste and inclusion of more zinc-rich foods in the diet, such as seafood, whole grain products, and milk, might improve the taste and appeal of foods. In addition, a small amount of a strongly flavored food at the beginning of a meal can stimulate tastebuds, saliva flow, and interest in eating. The addition of more spices during cooking and at the table can improve the flavor of foods. An attractive table-setting and appetizing appearance and texture of food can also improve a person's appetite.[176]

Weight Control

Maintenance of a normal body weight helps prevent high blood pressure, diabetes, cancer, gallbladder disease, arthritis, and cardiovascular disease.[31] Over one-half of elderly women and nearly two-fifths of elderly men are obese.[18,33] Overweight people are less active and show reduced physical fitness, stamina, energy, and mental health. Underweight, on the other hand, also shortens life and is associated with malnutrition.[33]

Moderate exercise and a nutritious diet are the healthiest ways to lose weight. Activity increases metabolism and burns calories. Modest reduction in calories can help an individual lose fat weight, especially when combined with exercise.

Diets below 1,000 calories are ineffective for permanent weight loss. They slow metabolism, reduce burning of calories, and the weight lost is muscle rather than fat.[178] A safe rate of weight loss is two to three pounds a week. More than this means muscle and fluid rather than fat is lost and the weight will be hard to keep off. Losing and regaining the same 10 or 15 pounds is less healthy than maintenance of the extra weight.[179,180] *(Table 5)*

Table 5 Simple Menu For Weight Reduction (1,200 Calories)

Breakfast	**Lunch**
Prune juice, ¼ cup	Lean roast beef, 3 oz
Cereal, fortified, ¾ cup	Carrots, ½ cup
Nonfat milk, 8 oz	Rice, ½ cup
Whole wheat toast, 1 slice	Fruit (fresh orange), 1 small
Tea	Margarine, 1 tsp
	Coffee
Dinner	**Snack**
Baked chicken, 3 oz	Cantaloupe, ¼ medium
Cottage cheese, ½ cup	Nonfat milk, 8 oz
Tomato	
Lettuce	
Whole wheat bread, 1 slice	
Margarine, 1 tsp	
Fruit salad, ½ cup	

4
Medications And Nutrition

The elderly are the single largest users of medication in the United States and account for 25% of all drug purchases.[181] Over 80% of the elderly population take more than two medications each day.[182] Older adults are at high risk for nutritional problems. Frequent use of medications for chronic disease and minor complaints adds to the potential for nutrient deficiencies. As a person ages, medications are not metabolized as well and vulnerability to side effects increases.[183] The use of several medications at once compounds the risk for nutritional deficiencies. Errors in dose can more easily occur in seniors medicating themselves with several drugs.[184]

Drugs interact with nutrition in the following ways:

1. Food can increase or decrease absorption of drugs,
2. Components of the diet change the rate of drug use in the body,
3. Drugs interfere with nutrient pathways, increase excretion, and change nutrient needs, and
4. Drugs affect appetite, taste, and food intake.

Antihistamines, steroids, tranquilizers, and antidepressants can increase appetite and lead to weight gain. Several drugs, including alcohol and amphetamines, lower appetite and might lead to malnutrition.[185] Digitalis and cancer drugs cause nausea and vomiting. D-penicillamine used to treat rheumatoid arthritis can lead to loss of taste[186], as can diuretics, antibiotics, anticancer drugs, and drugs used to treat Parkinson's disease and hypertension. Unpleasant taste changes might result in too little food intake and malnutrition.

Drugs that interfere with absorption of vitamins, such as colchicine, can impair vitamin B_{12} absorption and might lead to anemia.[187] Alcohol interferes with thiamin and folic acid absorption, which increases nerve problems and anemia.[188] Laxatives can produce deficiencies of fat-soluble vitamins. The antibiotic neomycin has the same effect.[188]

Other drugs lead to mineral depletion. Alcohol and some diuretics cause excretion of potassium, zinc, and magnesium. Regular use of aspirin causes the stomach to bleed, leading to iron deficiency and anemia.[187] Antacids can produce phosphate deficiency, which leads to severe muscle weakness and convulsions.[185]

There are just a few of the hundreds of drug-nutrient interactions. (See PRESCRIPTION DRUGS AND NUTRITION, published by Health Media of America, Inc.)

5 Nutrition And Aging

Studies on centenarians show that a long life is associated with physical activity, close family ties, and sensible diets of fresh fruits and vegetables, whole grains, and little meat.[189,190]

The consumption of a low-calorie diet also might improve chances for longevity.[191-192] The earlier in life this type of diet is started, the longer the life.[192] A diet low, but adequate, in protein and high in complex carbohydrates such as fruits, vegetables, and whole grain breads and cereals also might extend life.[193]

Nutrition, health, and aging are intimately connected. Chronic illness is now the cause of 80% of deaths.[194,195] Dietary habits and weight control are an effective and essential means to prevent cancer, heart disease, osteoporosis, diabetes, and high blood pressure. A diet low in total fat, saturated fat, sugar, alcohol, and sodium and high in fiber and all nutrients is needed, with particular emphasis on adequate intake of vitamins A, E, C and D and the minerals calcium, chromium, and selenium.

The B vitamins are crucial to a healthy nervous system and alert mind. Protein, calories, and a wide range of vitamins and minerals keep the immune system strong. Chronic diseases also create new nutrient demands that can accelerate aging. Colds, infections, acute illnesses, and accidents require optimal nutrition in order to minimize sickness.[194]

Exercise is essential to a healthy, long life. The advise to "use it or lose it" applies to the health of the heart, lungs, and circulatory system.[196] Rather than wearing out the body, regular physical activity prevents it from deteriorating. Exercise also helps control chronic stress, which takes its toll on physical and mental health and increases risk of heart disease, cancer, high blood pressure, and diabetes.

Aging is not a disease; it is a lifelong process and a natural part of the beauty and joy of life.

Appendix
The Nutrition Marketplace

Shopping And Cooking Tips

The following are some ideas to help overcome common problems in shopping and preparing food. Shopping for one or two:

- Buy small packages of items. Though sometimes more expensive, it is better than buying larger packages that spoil.
- Buy small amounts of fresh produce. Buy some that are ripe and some that will ripen in a day or two. Buy produce in season to avoid higher cost.
- Large bags of frozen vegetables are more economical than smaller packages. Remove what you need, seal, and return the bag to the freezer.
- When selecting whole grain breads, read the label; only those varieties that state "100% whole wheat" are guaranteed to contain whole wheat flour as the primary ingredient.
- Shop at a store that carries staples, such as rice, beans, or biscuit mixes in bulk and purchase only as much as is needed.
- Use dried skim milk powder in cooking. It is cheaper than fresh milk, stores longer, and works well for many uses. Sprinkle it into soups, sauces, and other dishes to boost calcium intake.
- Read ingredients labels on packaged foods. Avoid any foods that show fat or sugar as the first or

second ingredient or that list different types of fat or sweeteners more than once.

- Ask for individual servings of lean meat to be wrapped rather than purchasing large packages of meat. If large packages of lean meat are purchased divide them into smaller portions, rewrap with foil or plastic, and store in the freezer. Loaves of bread also can be frozen.
- Keep staples on hand, such as canned tuna, canned vegetables, fruit juices, and cereal to avoid frequent shopping trips. *(Table 6, Page 49)*

How To Simplify Cooking:

- When cooking casseroles, soups, and stews, double the recipe and store one batch in the freezer or divide the dish into individual portions for easy reheating at a later time.
- Use leftover vegetables and meat in soup or stew.
- Sit down while preparing foods. Have a chair or stool of suitable height for the counters and stove.
- Keep pots and utensils within easy reach. If the cupboards are too low or too high for easy reaching, hang things on hooks or nails on the walls.
- Heat leftovers in one pan for easy clean-up.
- Save aluminum trays from TV dinners to make homemade nutritious versions from leftovers.

When Choosing A Vitamin-Mineral Supplement Program:

- Choose a supplement program that provides the vitamins and minerals in amounts close to the USRDA. The amount of a nutrient is expressed as a percent on the label. If the nutrient is at the level of the USRDA it will say "100%."

Table 6 Shopping Wisely

Unwise Choice	Better Choice
Whole milk, sour cream, cream, nondairy creamers made with coconut or palm oil.	Low-fat or nonfat milk, evaporated nonfat milk.
Cream cheese, cheddar, and other whole milk cheeses.	Neufchatel cheese, low-fat cottage cheese, ricotta cheese, farmer cheese, part skim mozzarella.
Whole milk, fruited yogurt.	Plain, low-fat yogurt (add your own fruit).
Vegetables in sauces, canned vegetables, fruits in syrup, sweetened fruit juices.	Plain, fresh, or frozen vegetables, fresh or unsweetened fruits and juices, dried fruits.
Ready-to-eat muffins, waffles, quick breads, donuts, sugar-coated or high sugar cereals, baking mixes, white rice.	Whole grain breads, rolls, crackers, flours and pastas, unsweetened whole grain cereals (oatmeal, shredded wheat, grape nuts, cheerios, etc), brown rice.
Beef with visible fat marbling, corned beef, bacon, sausage, breaded frozen seafood, tuna packed in oil, hot dogs, luncheon meats.	Chicken, turkey, plain fish, tuna packed in water, dry beans and peas, lean meat cuts (bottom round, flank steak, lean hamburger).
Peanut butter with hydrogenated oil added, salted nuts.	Unsalted "old-fashioned" peanut butter, unsalted raw nuts.
Ice cream, pastries, cakes, cookies.	Ice milk, fruit.
Lard, coconut oil, palm, oil, hydrogenated or partially hydrogenated shortening, hard margarines.	Butter, safflower oil, corn oil, cornflower seed oil, soy oil, soft margarines, (USE ALL FATS & OILS SPARINGLY).

References

1. Williams E, Caliendo M: *Nutrition Principles, Issues, and Applications.* New York, McGraw-Hill Book Company, 1984, pp 458-461.
2. *Statistical Abstracts of the United States.* US Dept of Commerce, Bureau of Census, 1980.
3. Hamilton E, Whitney E: *Understanding Nutrition.* St Paul, West Publishing Co, 1984, pp 27,145,381,387.
4. Roe D: *Geriatric Nutrition.* Englewood Cliffs, Prentice-Hall Inc, 1983, pp 11-24.
5. Williams E, Caliendo M: *Nutrition Principles, Issues, and Applications.* New York, McGraw Book Co, 1984, p 549.
6. Hamilton E, Whitney E: *Understanding Nutrition.* St Paul, West Publishing Co, 1984, p 461.
7. Schlenker E, Feurig J, Stone L: Nutrition and health of older people, in Labuza R, Sloan A: *Contemporary Nutrition Controversies.* St Paul, West Publishing Co, 1979, pp 301-313.
8. Hamilton E, Whitney E: *Understanding Nutrition.* St Paul, West Publishing Co, 1984. pp 550-562.
9. Watkins D: Nutrition For the Aging and the Aged, in Goodhart R, Shils M (eds), *Modern Nutrition in Health and Disease,* ed 5, Philadelphia, Lea and Febiger, 1973, pp 781-813.
10. Busse E: How mind, body, and environment influence nutrition in the elderly. *Postgrad Med* 1978; 63:118-125.
11. Nutritional Problems of the Elderly. Feeherry M, Reiff T, Shank R, Van Itallie T, White P (Discussants). *Dialog Nutr* 1977; 2(3).
12. Schneider E, Eugenia M, Vining M, et al: Recommended dietary allowances and the health of the elderly. *N Eng J Med* 1986; 314:157-160.
13. Roe D: *Geriatric Nutrition.* Englewood Cliffs, Prentice-Hall Inc, 1983, pp 11-24.
14. Kelley L, Ohlson M, Harper L: Food selection and well-being of aging women. *J Am Diet A* 1957; 33:466.
15. Chope H: Relation of nutrition to health in aging persons. *Calif Med* 1954; 81:335.

16. Garrison R, Somer E: *The Nutrition Desk Reference.* New Canaan, Conn, Keats Publishing Co, 1985, pp 116-123.
17. Roe D: *Geriatric Nutrition.* Englewood Cliffs, Prentice-Hall Inc, 1983, pp 83-84.
18. *Ten-State Nutrition Survey,* 1968-1970: V. Dietary DHEW, Publ No (HSM)72-1833. Atlanta: US Department of Health, Education and Welfare, Center For Disease Control 1972.
19. Preliminary findings of the First Health and Nutrition Examination Survey, US 1971-1972. *Dietary Intake and Biochemical Findings.* Washington DC, US Government Printing Office 1974, DHEW Publ No (HRA)74-1219-1.
20. *Nutrition Canada National Survey,* 1979-1972. Report by Nutrition Canada to the Dept of National Health and Welfare. Ottawa, Information Canada 1973.
21. Shank R: Nutritional characteristics of the elderly-an overview, in Rockstein M, Sussman M (eds), *Nutrition, Longevity and Aging.* New York, Academic Press 1976, pp 9-28.
22. Yearick E, Wang M, Pisias S: Nutritional status of the elderly: Dietary and biochemical findings. *J Gerontol* 1980; 35:663-671.
23. *USDA Household Food Consumption Survey.* Family Economics Research Group, Science and Education Administration, US Dept of Agriculture, Hyattsville, MD, 20782, 1980.
24. Roland D: Nutrition in adulthood and the later years, in Krause M, Mahan L: *Food, Nutrition, and Diet Therapy,* ed 7. WB Saunders Co, Philadelphia 1984, pp 319-333.
25. Anderson R, Kozlovsky A: Chromium intake, absorption and excretion of subjects consuming self-selected diets. *Am J Clin Nutr* 1985; 42: 1177-1183.
26. Sandstead H: Zinc nutrition in the United States. *Am J Clin Nutr* 1973; 26:1251.
27. Roe D: *Geriatric Nutrition.* Englewood Cliffs, Prentice-Hall Inc, 1983, pp 63-69.
28. Craig G, Elliot C, Hughes K: Masked vitamin B_{12} and folate deficiency in the elderly. *Br J Nutr* 1985; 54:613-619.

29. MacLaughlin J, Holick M: Aging decreases the capacity of human skin to produce vitamin D3. *J Clin Invest* 1985; 76:1536-1538.
30. Koehler H, Lee H, Jacobsen M: Tocopherols in canned entrees and vended sandwiches. *J Am Diet Assoc* 1977; 70:616-620.
31. *Dietary Goals for the United States,* ed 2. Select Committee on Nutrition and Human Needs United States Senate, December 1977. Washington DC, US Government Printing Office, Publ No 052-070-04376-8.
32. *Recommended Dietary Allowances,* ed 9. Committee on Dietary Allowances, Food and Nutrition Board, National Research Council. Washington DC, National Academy of Sciences 1980, pp 16-26.
33. Chenault A: *Nutrition and Health.* New York, Holt, Rinehart and Winston 1984, pp 658-664.
34. Kirk J, Chieffi M: Hypovitaminemia A: Effect of vitamin A administration on plasma vitamin A concentration, conjunctival changes, dark adaptation and toad skin. *Am J Clin Nutr* 1952; 1:37.
35. Rafsky H: Special nutritional problems of the aged. *Symposium on Problems of Gerontology.* New York, National Vitamin Foundation, 1954.
36. Girdwood R: Deficiencies of folic acid and vitamin B_{12} in the elderly in, Exton-Smith A, Scott D (eds): *Vitamins in the Elderly,* Bristol, England, John Wright and Sons, Ltd. 1968.
37. Evans D: Haematological aspects of iron deficiency in the elderly. Symposium on Iron, Anemia, and Old Age. *Geront Clin* 1971; 13:12-30.
38. Garrison R, Somer E: *The Nutrition Desk Reference.* New Canaan, Conn, Keats Publishing Co, 1985, pp 213-215.
39. Garn S: The earlier gain and later loss of cortical bone in nutritional perspective, Springfield, Illinois, Thomas, 1970, p 86-96.
40. Smith R, Rizek J: Epidemiologic studies of osteoporosis in women of Puerto Rico and southeastern Michigan with special reference to age, race, national origin, and to other related or associated findings. *Clin Orthopaed Related Res* 1966; 45:31.

41. Garn S: The course of bone gain and the phases of bone loss. *Orthopedic Clin N Am* 1972; 3:503.
42. Burkitt D: Relationships between diseases and their etiological significance. *Am J Clin Nutr* 1977; 30:262-267.
43. Kelsay J: A review of research on effects of fiber intake. *Am J Clin Nutr* 1978; 31:142.
44. Rheinhold J: Decreased absorption of calcium, magnesium, zinc and phosphorus by humans due to increased fiber and phosphorus consumption. *J Nutr* 1976; 106:493.
45. Chenault A: *Nutrition and Health.* New York, Holt, Rinehart and Winston 1984, p 185.
46. Garrison R, Somer E: *The Nutrition Desk Reference.* New Canaan, Conn, Keats Publishing Co, 1985, p 189-190.
47. Roe D: Problems of nutrition in the aged. *J Am Ger Soc* 1973; 21:363-367.
48. Liebman B: Water, water everywhere. *Nutrition Action* 1982; 9:14.
49. Leiber C: Alcohol-nutrient interaction. *Contemporary Nutrition* 1983; 8:1-2.
50. Olson R: Nutrition and alcoholism, in Goodhart R, Shils M (eds): *Modern Nutrition in Health and Disease,* ed 5. Philadelphia: Lea and Febiger 1973, pp 1037-1050.
51. Harant A, Goldberger J: Treatment of anemia in the aged: A common problem and challenge. *J Am Ger Soc* 1975; 23:127-131.
52. Garry P, Goodwin J, Hunt W: Folate and vitamin B_{12} status in a healthy elderly population. *J Am Ger Soc* 1984; 32:719-726.
53. Helliwel M, Coombes E, Moody B, et al; Nutritional-status in rheumatoid arthritis (meeting abstract). *Br J Rheum* 1984; 23(2):117.
54. Helliwell M, Coombes E, Moody B, et al: Nutritional status in patients with rheumatoid arthritis. *Ann Rheum D* 1984; 43:386-390.
55. Reid D, Kennedy J, Smith M, et al: Total body calcium in rheumatoid arthritis: Effects of disease activity and corticosteroid treatment. *Br Med J* 1982; 285:330.

56. Williams S: *Nutrition and Diet Therapy,* ed 5. St. Louis, Times Mirror/Mosby College Publishing 1985, pp 656-606.
57. Blake D, Hall N, Treby D, et al: Protection against superoxide and hydrogen peroxide in synovial fluid from rheumatoid patients. *Clin Sci* 1981; 61:483-486.
58. Gough K, McCarthy C, Read A, et al: Folic acid deficiency in rheumatoid arthrtis. *Br Med J* 1964; 1:212-217.
59. Maddison P, Bacon P: Vitamin D deficiency, spontaneous fractures and osteopenia in rheumatoid arthritis. *Br Med J* 1974; 4:433-435.
60. Sanderson C, Davis R, Bayliss E: Serum pyridoxal in patients with rheumatoid arthritis. *Ann Rheum Dis* 1976; 35:177.
61. Bayles T: Nutrition in disease of the bones and joints, in Goodhart R, Shils M (eds): *Modern Nutrition in Health and Disease.* Philadelphia, Lea and Febiger 1973, pp 919-923.
62. Munthe E, Aaseth J: Treatment of rheumatic arthritis with selenium and vitamin E. *Scan J Rheum* 1984; S53:103.
63. UK, General Practitioner Research Group: Calcium pantothenate in arthritis conditions. *Practitioner* 1980; 224:208-211.
64. Chandra R, Tejpar S: Diet and immunocompetence. *Int J Imm* 1983; 5:175-180.
65. Michalek A, Kremer J, Bigaouet J, et al: Eicosapentaenoic acid (EPA) supplementation in rhematoid-arthritis (RA). *Am J Clin Nutr* 1985; 41:871.
66. Aspinall R, Cammarata P: Effect of prostaglandin E_2 on adjuvant arthritis. *Nature* 1969; 224:1320-1321.
67. Zurier R, Qualiata F: Effect of prostaglandin E_1 on adjuvant arthritis. *Nature* 1971; 234:304-305.
68. Denko C: Modification of adjuvant inflammation in rats deficient in essential fatty acids. *Agents Actions* 1976; 6:636-641.
69. Panush R, Carter R, Katz P, et al: Diet therapy for rheumatoid arthritis. *Arthritis Rheum* 1983; 26:462-471.
70. Podell R: Nutritional treatment of rheumatoid arthritis-can alterations in fat intake affect disease course? *Postgrad Med* 1985; 77:65.

71. Prickett J, Robinson D, Steinbert A: Dietary enrichment with the polyunsaturated fatty acid eicosapentaenoic acid prevents proteinuria and prolongs survival in NZB and NZW F1 mice. *J Clin Invest* 1981; 68:556-559.
72. Machty I, Ouaknine L: Tocopherol in osteoarthritis: A controlled pilot study. *J Am Ger Soc* 1978; 26:328-330.
73. Kamimura M: Anti-inflammatory activity of vitamin E. *Jap Med News* 1973; 88:13.
74. Wallace S: Gout and hypertension. *Arth Rheum* 1975; 18(supp):721.
75. Gibson T: A controlled study of diet in patients with gout. *Ann Rheum Dis* 1983; 42:123.
76. Stanbury J, Wyngaarden J, Frederickson D: *The Metabolic Basis of Inherited Disease,* ed 4. New York, McGraw-Hill 1978, pp 942.
77. Schaefer A: Nutrition problems of the elderly. *Nutrition News* 1980; 43:9-10.
78. Reynolds H, Preece J, Bailey J, et al: Folate deficiency in depressive illness. *Br J Psych* 1970; 117:287-289.
79. Holsboen F, Benkert O, Meier L, et al: Combined estradiol and vitamin B_6 treatment in women with major depression (letter). *Am J Psych* 1985; 142:658.
80. Baar W: Pyridoxine supplements in the premenstrual syndrome. *Practitioner* 1984; 228:425-427.
81. Groves P, Schlesinger K: *Introduction to Biological Psychology,* ed 2. Dubuque, William C Brown Co, 1982, pp 133,468,579-582.
82. Kreiger D, Hughes, J (eds): *Neuroendocrinology.* Sunderland MA, Sinauer Associates 1982, p 167-176.
83. Vitamin B_6 toxicity: A new megavitamin syndrome. *Nutr Rev* 1984; 42:44-46.
84. Pollet P, Leathwood P: The influence of tryptophan on sleep in man. *Int J Vit Nutr Res* 1983; 53:223.
85. Hartmann E, Grerenwald D: *Progress in Tryptophan and Serotonin Research.* New York, Walter de Gruyter and Co, 1984, p 297.
86. Marcus, J, Hetzberg, Freedman M: Vitamin B_{12} and transcobalamin II levels in memory functioning in the elderly (meeting abstract). *Gerontol* 1985; 25:158.
87. Wurtman R, Bluzstajn J, Maire J: "Autocannibalism" of choline-containing membrane phospholipids

in the pathogenesis of Alzheimer's disease: A hypothesis. *Neurochem I* 1985; 7:369-372.

88. King R, Sharp J, Boura A: Aluminum, choline transportation and Alzheimers disease (letter). *Med J Aust* 1983; 2:606-607.
89. Heath H: Progress against osteoporosis (editorial). *Ann Int Med* 1983; 98:1011-1013.
90. Mazess E, Cameron J: Bone mineral content in normal U.S. whites, in *International Conference on Bone Mineral Measurement,* Chicago, US DHEW, 1973, pp 228-238.
91. Jensen G, Christiansen C, Boesen J, et al: Epidemiology of postmenopausal spinal and long bone fractures. *Clin Orthop* 1982; 166:75-81.
92. Cohn S, Vaswani A, Zanzi I, et al: Effect of aging on bone mass in adult women. *Am J Physiol* 1976; 230:143-148.
93. Jowsey J: Osteoporosis. Its nature and the role of diet. *Postgrad Med* 1976; 60:75-79.
94. Riggs B: Effect of the fluoride/calcium regimen on vertebral fracture occurrence in postmenopausal osteoporosis. *N Engl J Med* 1982; 306:446.
95. Recker R: Osteoporosis. *Contemporary Nutrition* 1983; 8:1-2.
96. Recker R, Saville P, Heaney R: Effect of estrogens and calcium carbonate on bone loss in postmenopausal women. *Ann Int Med* 1977; 87:649.
97. Albanese A: Osteoporosis. *Cont Nutr* 1977; 2:1-2.
98. Albanese A, Lorenze E, Edelson A, et al: Effects of calcium supplements and estrogen replacement therapy on bone loss of postmenopausal women. *Nut Rep Internat* 1981; 24:403-414.
99. Check W: Add exercise to calcium in osteoporosis prevention. *JAMA* 1982; 247:1108.
100. Avioli L: Postmenopausal osteoporosis: Prevention versus cure. *Fed Proc* 1981; 40:2418-2422.
101. Gallagher J, Riggs B, Eisman J, et al: Intestinal calcium absorption and serum vitamin D metabolites in normal subjects and osteoporotic patients. *J Clin Invest* 1979; 64:729-736.

102. Albanese A, Edelson A, Lorenze E, et al: Problems of bone health in elderly. *NY State J Med* 1975; 75:326-336.
103. Nordin B, Horsman A, Crilly A: Treatment of spinal osteoporosis in postmenopausal women. *Br Med J* 1980; Feb 16:451-454.
104. Shiraki M, Orimo H, Ito H, et al: Long-term treatment of postmenopausal osteoporosis with active vitamin D_3, 1-alpha-hydroxycholecalciferol (1-alpha-OHD3) and 1,24 dihydroxycholecalciferol (1,24(OH)2D3). *Endocr Jpn* 1985; 32:305-315.
105. Pittet P, Davie M, Lawson D: Role of nutrition in the development of osteomalacia in the elderly. *Nutr Met* 1979; 23:109-116.
106. Tsai K, Heath H, Kumar R, et al: Impaired vitamin D metabolism with aging in women-possible role in pathogenesis of senile osteoporosis (meeting abstract). *Mayo Clinic and Mayo Foundation* 1984; 12:A411.
107. Buysschaert M, Lejeune D, Esselinck W, et al: Treatment of postmenopausal osteoporosis with vitamin D and severe hypercalcemia. *Act Clin B* 1984; 39:171-173.
108. White M, Martin R, Yeater R, et al: The effects of exercise on the bones of postmenopausal women. *Int Ortop* 1984; 7:209-214.
109. *Diet, Nutrition and Cancer.* Committee on Diet, Nutrition and Cancer, National Research Council, National Academy of Sciences. Washington DC, National Academy Press 1982.
110. Wynder E: The dietary environment and cancer. *J Am Diet A*ssoc 1977; 71:385-392.
111. Hirayama T: Changing patterns of cancer in Japan with special reference to the decrease in stomach cancer mortality, in Healt H, Watson J, Winston J (eds), *Origins of Human Cancer.* Book A, Incidence of Cancer in Humans. Cold Spring Harbor, New York, Cold Spring Harbor Laboratory 1977.
112. Tuyns A: Protective effect of citrus fruit on esophageal cancer. *Nutr Cancer* 1983; 5:195-200.

113. Gordon J, Scrimshaw N: Infectious disease in the malnourished. *Med Clin No Amer* 1970; 54:1495-1508.
114. Tappel A: Where old age begins. *Nutr Today* 1967; 2:4.
115. Chow C: Nutritional influence on cellular antioxidant defense systems. *Am J Clin Nutr* 1979; 23:1066.
116. Prasad K, Edwards-Prasad J: Effects of tocopherol (Vitamin E) acid succinate on morphological alterations and growth inhibition in melanoma cells in culture. *Cancer Research* 1982; 42:550.
117. Capel I, Leach D, Dorell H: Vitamin E retards the lipoperoxidation resulting from anticancer drug administration. *Anticancer Research* 1983; 3:59.
118. Spallholz J: Selenium: What role in immunity and immune cytotoxicity? in Spallholz J, Martin J, Ganther H (eds), *Selenium in Biology and Medicine.* Westport Conn, AVI Publishers 1981, pp 103-117.
119. Sundstrom H, Yrjanhei E, Kauppila A: Low selenium concentration in patients with cervical or endometrial cancer. *Int J Gyn Obes* 1984; 22: 35-40.
120. Shamberger R, Tytkos S, Willis C: Antioxidants and cancer. *Arch Environ Health* 1976; 31:231-235.
121. Yang, G, Wang S, Zhou R, et al: Endemic selenium intoxication of humans in China. *Am J Clin Nutr* 1983; 37:872.
122. MacLennan R, Da Costa J, Day N, et al: Shanmugaratnam K: Risk factors for lung cancer in Singapore Chinese, a population with high female incidence rates. *Int J Cancer* 1977; 20: 854-860.
123. Mettlin C, Graham S, Swanson M: Vitamin A and lung cancer. *J Nat Canc Inst* 1979; 62:1435-1438.
124. Bjelke E: Dietary vitamin A and human lung cancer. *Int J Cancer* 1975; 15:561-565.
125. Wald N, Idle M, Boreham J, et al: Low serum-vitamin-A and subsequent risk of cancer: Preliminary results of a prospective study. *Lancet* 1980; 2:813-815.
126. Kark J, Smith A, Switzer B, et al: Serum vitamin A (retinol) and cancer incidence in Evans County, Georgia. *J Nat Canc Inst* 1981; 66:7-16.

127. McCormick D, Burns F, Albert R: Inhibition of benzopyrene-induced mammary carcinogenesis by retinyl acetate. *J Nat Canc Inst* 1981; 66:559-564.
128. Beretti B, Grupper C, Edelson Y, et al: Aromatic retinoid in the treatment of multiple superficial basal cell carcinoma, arsenic keratosis and keratoacanthoma, in Orfanos C (ed), Retinoids: *Advances in Basic Research and Therapy* Berlin, New York, Springer-Verlag, 1981.
129. Haydey R, Reed M, Daubox L, et al: Treatment of keratoacanthomas with oral 13-cis-retinoic acid. *N Engl J Med* 1980; 303:560-562.
130. Hirayama T: Diet and Cancer. *Nutr Canc* 1979; 1:67-81.
131. Hamilton E, Whitney E: *Understanding Nutrition*. St Paul, West Publishing Co, 1984, pp 330-331.
132. *Recommended Dietary Allowances* 9 ed. Committee on Dietary Allowances, Food and Nutrition Board, National Research Council, Washington DC, National Academy of Sciences, 1980, p 59.
133. Harris W, Conner W, Inkles S, et al: Dietary omega-3 fatty acid prevent carbohydrate-induced hypertriglyceridemia. *Metabolism* 1984; 33:1016-1019.
134. Simons L, Hickie J, Balasubramaniam S: On the effects of dietary n-3 fatty acids (MaxEPA) on plasma lipids and lipoproteins in patients with hyperlipidaemia. *Atherosclerosis* 1985; 54: 75-88.
135. Chenault A: *Nutrition and Health*. New York, Holt, Rinehart and Winston 1984, p 171.
136. Altschul A, Grommet J: Sodium intake and sodium sensitivity. *Nutr Rev* 1980; 38:393-402.
137. Jacobs M, Leibman B: Dietary sodium and the risk of hypertension (correspondence). *N Eng J Med* 1980; 303:817-818.
138. McCarron D: Low serum concentration of ionized calcium in patients with hypertension. *N Engl J Med* 1982; 307:226-228.
139. Resnick L, Nicholson J, Laragh J: Outpatient therapy of essential hypertension with dietary calcium supplementation. *J Am College Card* 1984; 3:616.
140. Chenault A: *Nutrition and Health*. New York, Rinehart and Winston, 1984, p 402.

141. Rouse I, Beilin L, Armstrong B, et al: Vegetarian diet, blood pressure and cardiovascular risk. *Aust NZ J Med* 1984; 14:439-443.
142. Pusak P, Nissinen A, Pietinen P, et al: Dietary fat and human blood pressure (meeting abstract). *Circulation* 1985; 71:A417.
143. Iacano M: Reduction in blood pressure associated with high polyunsaturated fat diets that reduce blood cholesterol in man. *Prev Med* 1975; 4:426.
144. Judd J: Effects of diets varying in fat and P/S ratio on blood pressure in man. *Fed Proc* 1979; 38:387.
145. Comberg H: Hypotensive effect of dietary prostaglandin precursor in hypertensive man. Prostaglandins 1978; 15:193. 146. Pheir J: Aging and infection: A review. *J Chron Dis* 1979; 32:535-540.
147. Weksler M, Innes J, Goldstein G: The role of the thymus in the senescence of the immune response, in Singal S, Sinclair N, Stiller C (eds), *Aging and Immunity.* New York, Elsevier/North Holland, 1979, pp 165-172.
148. Bennet P: Diabetes in the elderly: Diagnosis and epidemiology. *Geriatrics* 1984; 39:37-41.
149. Kent S: Is diabetes a form of accelerated aging? *Geriatrics* 1976; 31:140,145,149-151
150. Gregerman R, Bierman E: Aging and Hormones. in Williams R (ed), *Textbook of Endocrinology.* Philadelphia, W B Saunders and Sons, 1981, pp 1192-1209.
151. Jarrett R, McCartney P, Keen H: The Bedford survey: Ten year mortality rates in newly diagnosed diabetics, borderline diabetics and normoglycemic controls and risk indices for coronary artery disease in borderline diabetics. *Diabetologia* 1983; 22:79-94.
152. Williams S: *Nutrition and Diet Therapy,* ed 5. St. Louis, Times Mirror/Mosby College Publishing, 1985, p 579.
153. Lipson L: *Diabetes Mellitus in the Elderly: Special Problems, Special Approaches.* Los Angeles: University of Southern California School of Medicine, 1985.
154. Lipson L, Lipson M: The therapeutic approach to the obese maturity-onset diabetic patient. *Arch Intern Med* 1984; 144:135-138.

155. Offenbacher E: Beneficial effect of chromium-rich yeast on glucose tolerance and blood lipids in elderly subjects. *Diabetes* 1980; 29:919-925.
156. Williams E, Caliendo M: *Nutrition Principles, Issues, and Applications.* New York, McGraw-Hill Book Company, 1984, p 74.
157. Hamilton E, Whitney E: *Understanding Nutrition.* St Paul, West Publishing Company, 1984, p 498.
158. Roe D: *Geriatric Nutrition.* Englewood Cliffs, Prentice-Hall Inc, 1983, p 151.
159. Kahin H: Laxatives: A last resort in chronic constipation. *Consultant* 1977:March; 25-27.
160. Chernow B, Castell O: Diet and heartburn. *JAMA* 1979; 241:2307-2308.
161. Ribakove B: Private enemies: *Gas. Health* 1983; 15:44.
162. Armstrong B, Doll R: Environmental factors and cancer incidence and mortality in different countries, with special reference to dietary practices. *Int J Cancer* 1975; 15:617.
163. Handler S: Dietary fiber-can it prevent colon diseases? *Postgrad Med* 1983; 73:301-307. 164. Garabran D, Peters J, Mack T, et al: Job activity in colon cancer risk. *Am J Epidem* 1984; 119:1005-1014.
165. Burkitt D: Epidemiology of cancer of the colon and rectum. *Cancer* 1971; 28:3-13.
166. Walker A, Burkitt D: Colon cancer epidemiology. *Semin Oncol* 1976; 3:4.
167. Reddy B, Cohen L, McCoy G, et al: Nutrition and its relation to cancer. *Adv Cancer Res* 1980; 32:237-345.
168. Shils M: Nutrition and neoplasia, in Goodhart R, Shils M (eds): *Modern Nutrition in Health and Disease* 6 ed. Philadelphia, Lea and Febiger, 1980, pp 1153-1192.
169. Trowell H: Definition of dietary fiber and hypothesis that it is a proctetive factor in certain diseases. *Am J Clin Nutr* 1976; 29:417-427.
170. Kaplan H: The oral cavity in geriatrics. *Geriatrics* 1971; 26:96-102.
171. Nizel A: Role of nutrition in the oral health of the aging patient. *Dent Clin N Am* 1976; 20:569-584.
172. Daniell H: Postmenopausal tooth loss. *Arch Intern Med* 1983; 143:1678-1682.

173. Anderson E: Eating patterns before and after dentures. *J Am Dent Soc* 1971; 58:421-426.
174. Kamath S: Taste acuity and aging. *Am J Clin Nutr* 1982; 36:766-775.
175. Schiffman S: Food recognition by the elderly. *J Gerontology* 1977; 32:586-592.
176. Schiffman S, Pasternak M: Decreased discrimination of food odors in the elderly. *J Gerontology* 1979; 34:73-79.
177. Schiffman S, Hornack K, Reilly D: Increased taste thresholds of amino acids with age. *Am J Clin Nutr* 1979; 32:1622-1627.
178. Madden C: What keeps obese persons obese? *Can Assoc Health Pys Ed Rec J* 1983; Jul-Aug:5-7.
179. Kohrs M: The prudent diet for the elderly. Presented at Stanford University School of Medicine, Palo Alto, Calif, 1980.
180. Andres R: Influence of obesity on longevity in the aged. *Adv Path* 1980; 7; 238-246.
181. Gibson R, Mueller J, Fisher C: Age differences in healthcare spending. Fiscal Year 1976. *Soc Sec Bull* 1977; 40:3-14.
182. Chien C, Townsend E, Townsend A: Substance use and abuse among the community elderly: The medical aspect. *Addict Dis* 1978; 3:357-372.
183. Dickerson J: Some adverse effects of drugs on nutrition. *Royal Soc Health J* 1978; 98:261-265.
184. Roe D: Drugs and nutrition in the geriatric patient. New York, Churchill Livingstone, 1984, pp 2-3.
185. Roe D: Interactions between drugs and nutrients. *Med Clin North Am* 1979; 63:985.
186. Roe D: *Geriatric Nutrition.* Englewood Cliffs, Prentice-Hall, Inc, 1983, p 84.
187. Williams S: *Nutrition and Diet Therapy,* ed 5. St Louis, Times Mirror/Mosby College Publishing, 1985, pp 513-515.
188. Rogers H: Food and medicine incompatibility. *Roy Soc Health* 1982; 102:1.
189. Murray M, Murray A: Diet and cardiovascular disease in centenarians of Hunza. *Arteriosclerosis* 1984; 4:546a.

190. Leaf A: Long-lived populations: Extreme old age. *J Am Geriatr Soc* 1982; 30:485-487.
191. Kahn A: Development, aging, and life duration: Effects of nutrient restriction. *J Am Clin Nutr* 1972; 25:822.
192. Ross M: Length of life and caloric intake. *Am J Clin Nutr* 1972; 25:834.
193. Rockstein M, Sussman M (eds), *Nutrition, Longevity and Aging.* New York Academic Press, 1976, pp 103-122.
194. Nutrition, Longevity, and Aging. *Dairy Council Digest* 1979; 50:19-22.
195. Upton A: Pathology, in Finch L, Hayflick L (eds), *The Biology of Aging.* New York, Van Nostrand Reinhold, 1977, pp 513-535.
196. Fries, J: Aging, natural death and the compression of morbidity. *N Engl J Med* 1980; 303:130-135.

Glossary

Achlorhydria: The lack of sufficient stomach acid to digest foods.

Anemia: A reduction in the number, size, or color of red blood cells; results in reduced oxygen carrying capacity of the blood.

Antioxidant: A compound that protects other compounds or tissues from oxygen by reacting with oxygen.

Autoimmunity: A condition where the immune system attacks organs or tissues of the body as if they were foreign bacteria or substances.

Beta Carotene: The form of vitamin A found in plant foods such as carrots and dark green leafy vegetables.

Bile: A fluid secreted by the liver into the intestines that mixes with other secretions to digest fats.

Calorie: A measurement of heat. In nutrition, calorie refers to the quantity of energy contained in foods.

Cancer: The uncontrolled growth of abnormal cells.

Carbohydrate: The starches and sugars in the diet.

Cardiovascular Disease: A disease of the heart and blood vessels often caused by an accumulation of cholesterol in the lining of the blood vessels.

Cholesterol: A type of fat found in foods from animal sources and produced in the liver. High levels of cholesterol in the blood are associated with the development of cardiovascular disease.

Colitis: Inflammation of the colon, which is the lower portion of the intestine.

CVD: See Cardiovascular Disease

Diabetes: A disorder in which the body's ability to use sugar is impaired because of inadequate production or utilization of the hormone insulin.

Diuretic: An agent that increases the flow of urine.

Diverticulosis: Disorder of the colon associated with inflammation and the development of pouches.

Eicosapentaenoic Acid (EPA): A type of unsaturated fat found in fish that might lower blood levels of cholesterol and the risk for developing cardiovascular disease.

Endometrial: The lining of the uterus.

Enzyme: Protein-like substances in the body that initiate and accelerate chemical reactions.

Esophagus: The passageway from the throat to the stomach.

Free Radical: A highly reactive compound derived from air pollution, radiation, cigarette smoke, or the incomplete breakdown of proteins and fats; reacts with fats in cell membranes and changes their shape or function.

Genetics: A branch of biology that studies heredity and biological variation.

Hemoglobin: The oxygen-carrying protein in red blood cells.

Hormone: A chemical substance produced by an organ, called an endocrine gland, that is released into the blood and transported to another organ or tissue, where it performs a specific action. Examples of hormones are estrogen, adrenalin, and insulin.

Hypertension: High blood pressure.

Immune System: A complex system of substances and tissues that protects the body from disease.

Lignin: A type of fiber found in some plant foods.

Metabolism: The sum total of all body processes, whereby the body converts foods into tissues and breaks down and repairs tissues and converts complex substances into simple ones for energy.

Obesity: Body weight more than 20% above desirable weight; excessive body fat.

Osteoporosis: Loss of calcium from the bones that results in porous, weak bones that are prone to fractures.

Prostaglandin: A group of hormone-like substances formed from fatty acids that have profound effects on the body, including contraction of smooth muscle and dilation or contraction of blood vessels

Prostate: An organ surrounding the neck of the bladder and beginning of the urethra in the male. This gland secretes a fluid that nourishes and hastens the movement of semen through the urethra.

Purine: Compounds in foods that might aggrevate the condition of gout. An example of a purine is uric acid.

Saturated Fat: A type of fat that is solid at room temperature and is found in foods from animal sources, hydrogenated vegetable oils, and coconut or palm oil. A diet high in saturated fats is linked to the development of cardiovascular disease and cancer.

Serotonin: A hormone-like substance produced in the brain that regulates mood, sleep, and numerous other body processes.

Stroke: Cerebrovascular accident caused by hemorrhage or a blood clot that blocks blood flow to a portion of the brain.

Tryptophan: An amino acid in the diet that the body uses to produce serotonin and the B vitamin niacin.

Unsaturated Fat: A type of fat that is liquid at room temperature and is primarily found in foods of plant sources such as vegetable oils, nuts, and seeds.

Index

W

Z

Notes